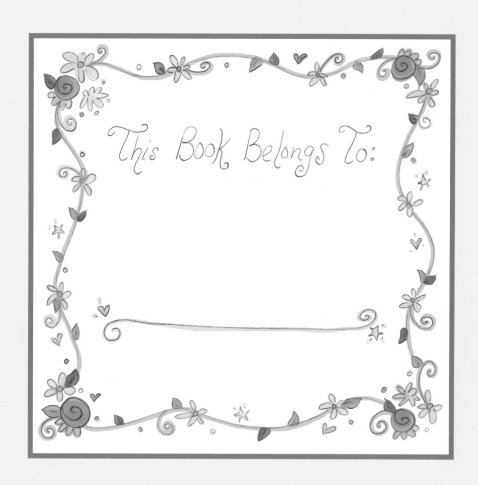

This Book Belongs To:

This book is dedicated to all the little princesses with food allergies.
Follow your dreams, they can come true.

And, to Sofia, my daughter, whose love of fairy tales inspired me to write this,
my daughter Isabella, my son Antonio, and my husband, Tony —
you light up my life!

And, thank you, Ms. Deirdre Humphrey, a special kindergarten teacher,
who, while teaching her class how to become authors,
succeeded in inspiring Sofia's mom too.

Kylie's Special Treat: A Food Allergy Fairy Tale, written by Letizia Barbetta, illustrated by Wendy Sefcik.
Published by Second Street Publishing LLC, Glenwood Landing, NY

QUANTITY DISCOUNTS ARE AVAILABLE TO YOUR EDUCATIONAL INSTITUTION, ORGANIZATION, OR COMPANY.

DISCLAIMER: The information contained herein is not intended to be a substitute for professional medical advice. Please seek the advice of your physician with regards to food allergies.

Cover Design by Wendy Sefcik. Interior design, storyboarding, and layout by Brian Taylor, Pneuma Books

Publisher's Cataloging-In-Publication Data

Barbetta, Letizia.
Kylie's special treat : a food allergy fairy tale / written by Letizia Barbetta ; illustrated by Wendy Sefcik. – 1st ed.

p. : col. ill. ; cm.

Summary: With some magical help, Kylie bakes a special treat for the prince that doesn't include any of the foods she's allergic to.
Kylie shows the reader how she manages her food allergies and goes on to live happily ever after.
Includes a simple baking recipe and food allergy tips and resources for adults.
Interest age level: 004-008.
ISBN: 978-1-935381-00-6

1. Food allergy in children–Juvenile fiction. 2. Food allergy in children–Fiction. 3. Fairy tales. I. Sefcik, Wendy. II. Title.

PZ7.B27 Kyl 2012
[Fic]

FIRST EDITION
Printed in the USA
20 19 18 17 16 15 14 13 12   01 02 03 04 05 06 07 08 09

Kylie's Special Treat

A Food Allergy Fairy Tale

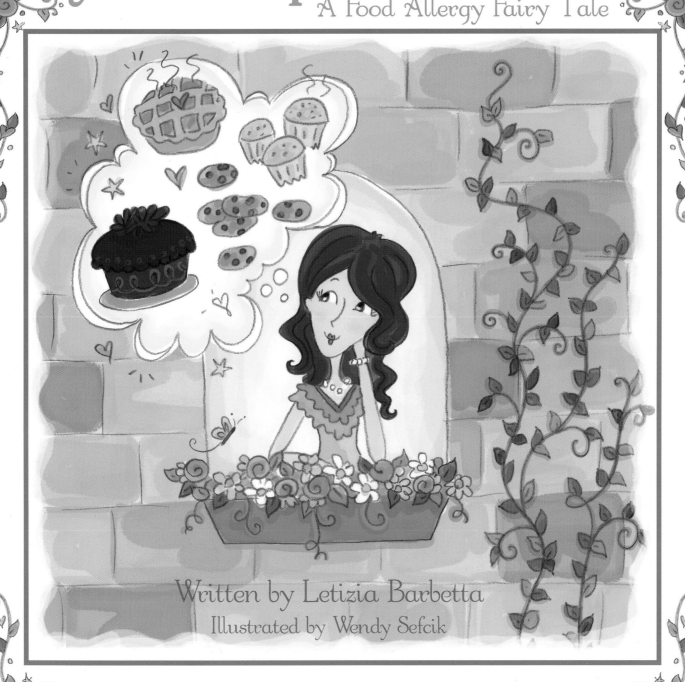

Written by Letizia Barbetta

Illustrated by Wendy Sefcik

Second Street Publishing, LLC

Gl̶... H̶...ling... N̶... York

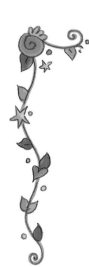
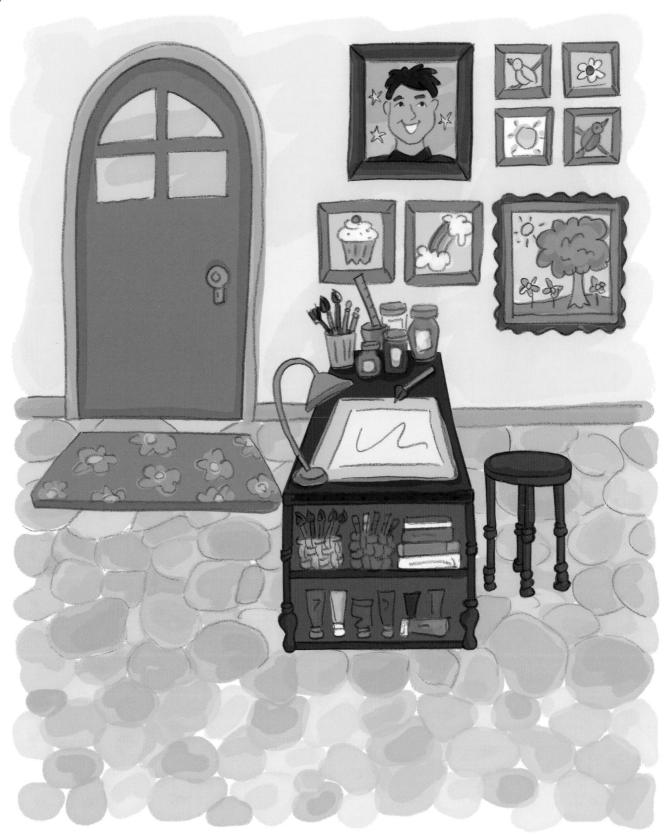

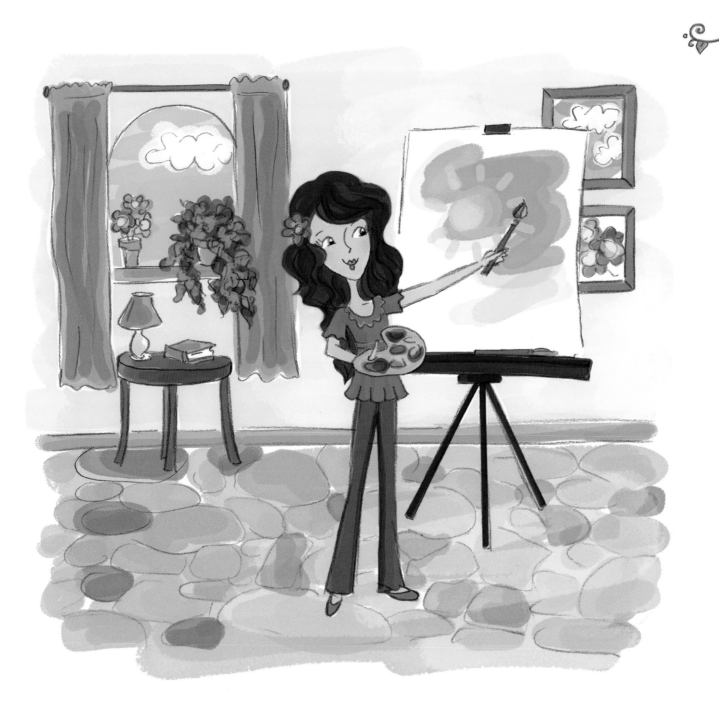

1

Once upon a time, there was a beautiful girl named
Kylie who loved to paint so much that she went
to art school, where she met Prince Steven.
Art school was over, but Kylie still dreamed of seeing
Prince Steven again and falling in love.

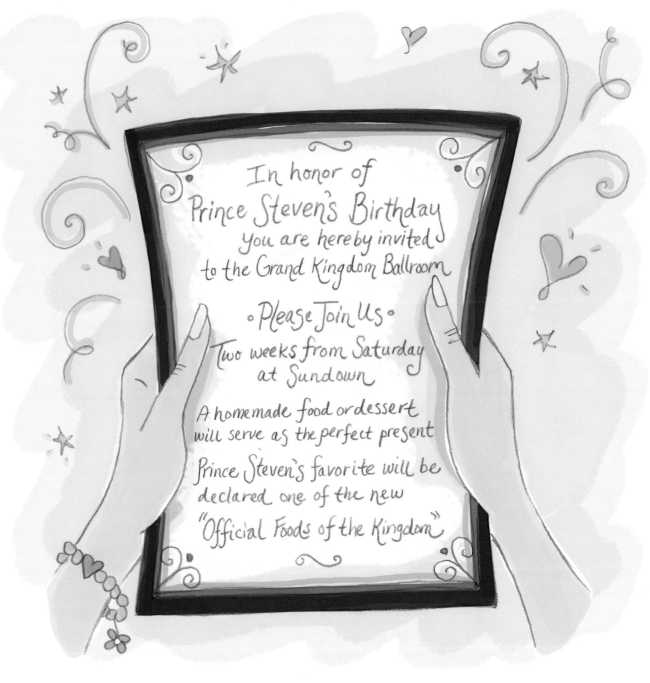

In honor of
Prince Steven's Birthday
you are hereby invited
to the Grand Kingdom Ballroom

• Please Join Us •

Two weeks from Saturday
at Sundown

A homemade food or dessert
will serve as the perfect present

Prince Steven's favorite will be
declared one of the new
"Official Foods of the Kingdom"

One afternoon while Kylie was painting,
she received an invitation to Prince Steven's ball.
"I'm going to see the prince again!" she said.
It didn't bother Kylie that she wouldn't be able to eat
any of the fancy foods at the ball.

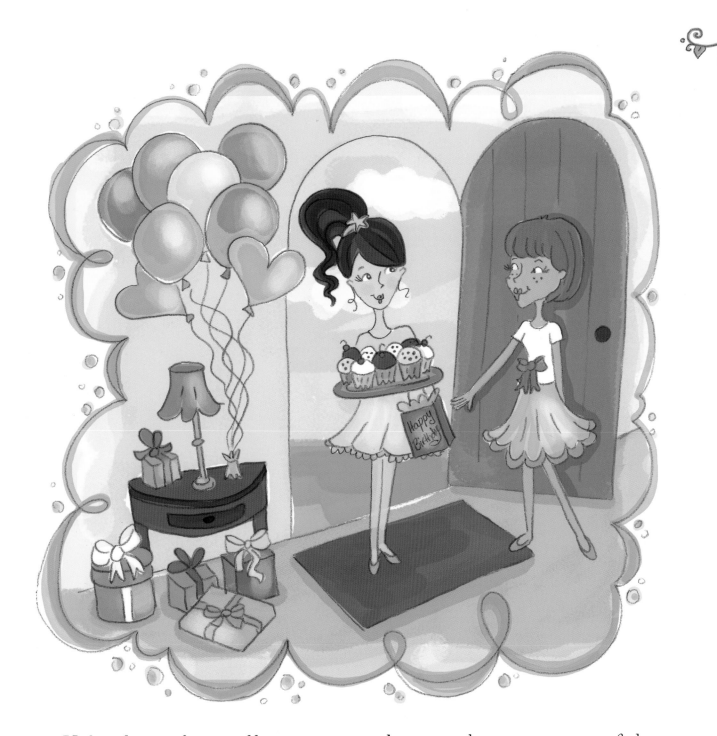

Kylie had food allergies and had to be extra careful
about the foods she ate, so she brought
her own food to parties. Some people said she was "special"
because of her allergies, but Kylie knew that
everybody was special in their own way.

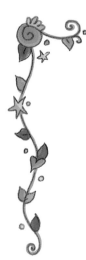

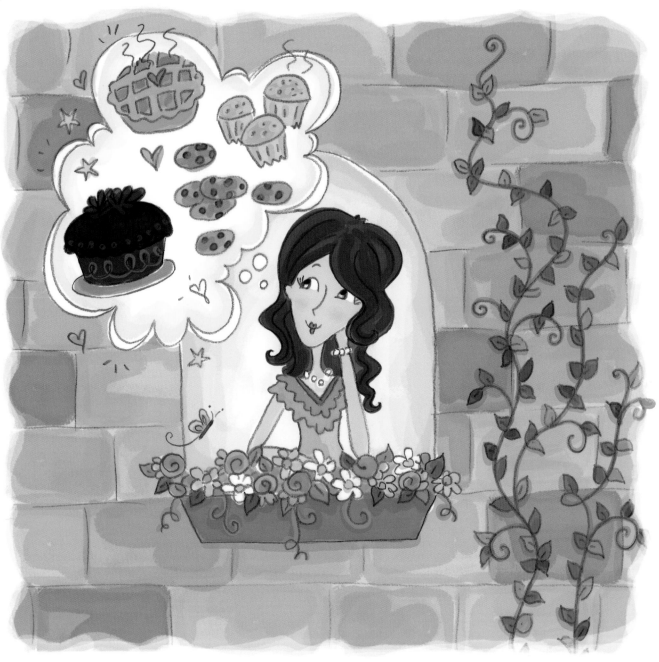

Kylie thought about what Prince Steven would like best.
"My dark chocolate velvet cake?
My moist banana muffins?
Sweet apple pie?
Or soft, chewy chocolate chip cookies?"

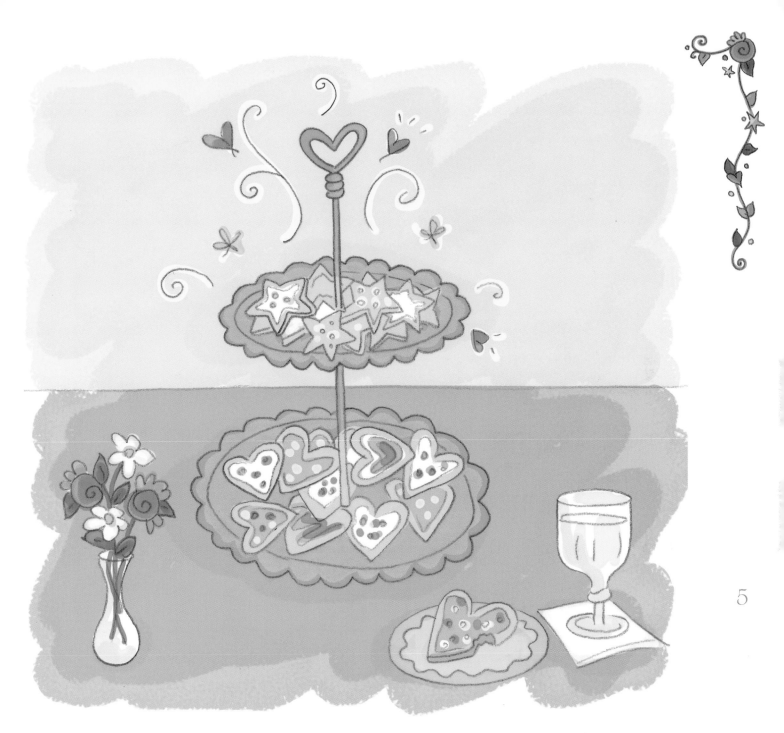

"Oh, I know!"
Kylie said excitedly.
"I'll make my favorite!
I will bake my super-delicious,
special sugar cookies!"

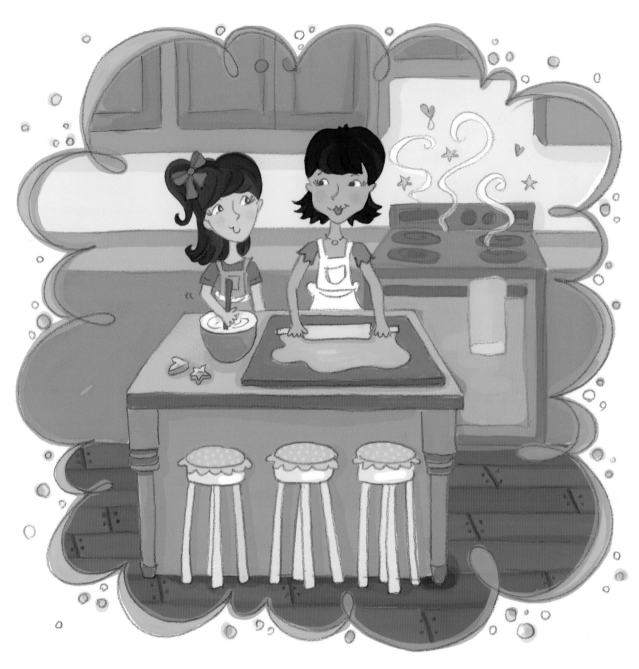

Kylie loved to bake.
When she was younger, she and her mom
would bake special treats for Kylie to eat at parties.
They were special because they were not made with any
of the foods she was allergic to.

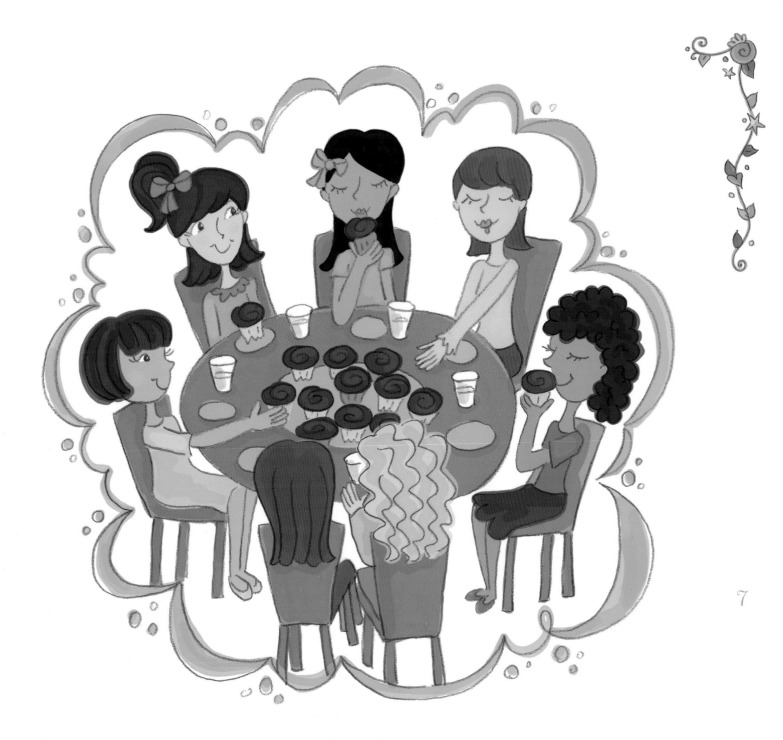

Sometimes Kylie brought extra
for her friends.
Everyone loved her desserts.
They were a special treat that
couldn't be found in any store.

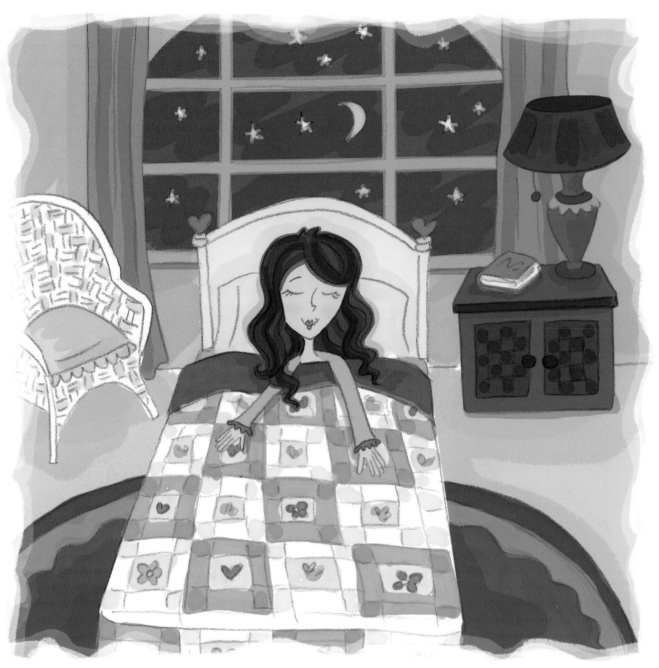

8

The night before the ball,
Kylie was so excited she could hardly sleep.
She wished over and over again,
"Please let me bake
the best sugar cookies ever!"

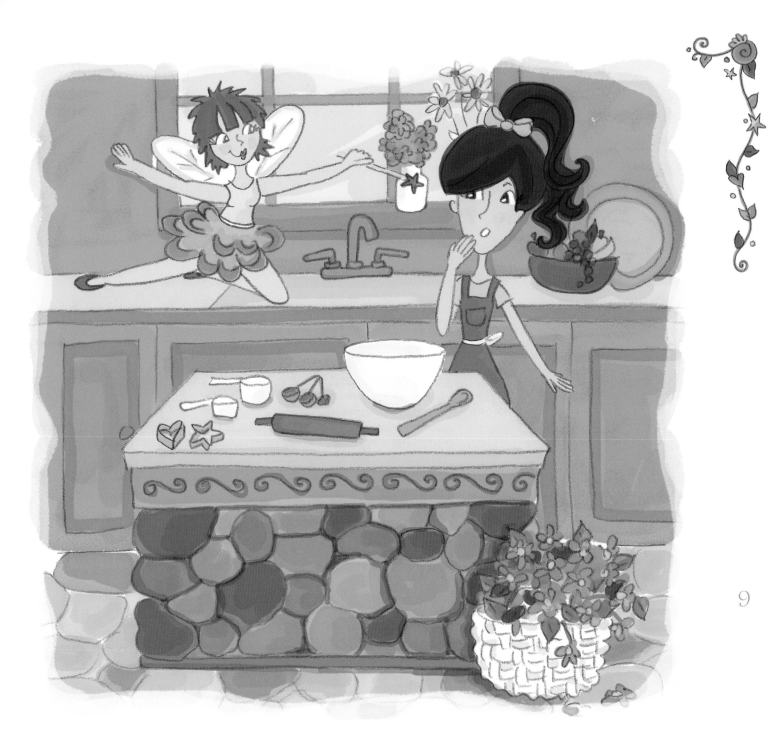

The next morning
when Kylie was putting on her apron for baking...
POOF, a fairy appeared.
"Are you my fairy godmother?" Kylie asked.
"No, sweetie, I'm the Food Fairy," said the flying lady,

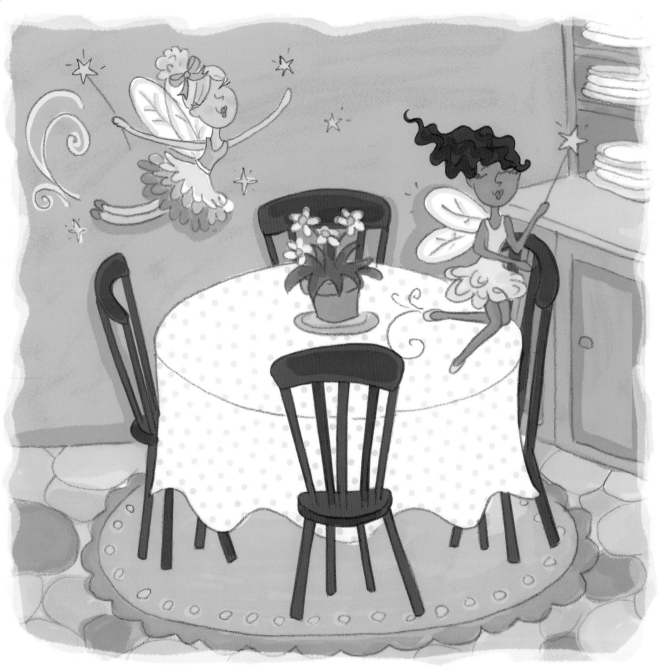

"and these are my baking fairies.
We're here to make sure you make
the best-tasting cookies—
just as you wished last night.
All you need is some milk, eggs, nuts..."

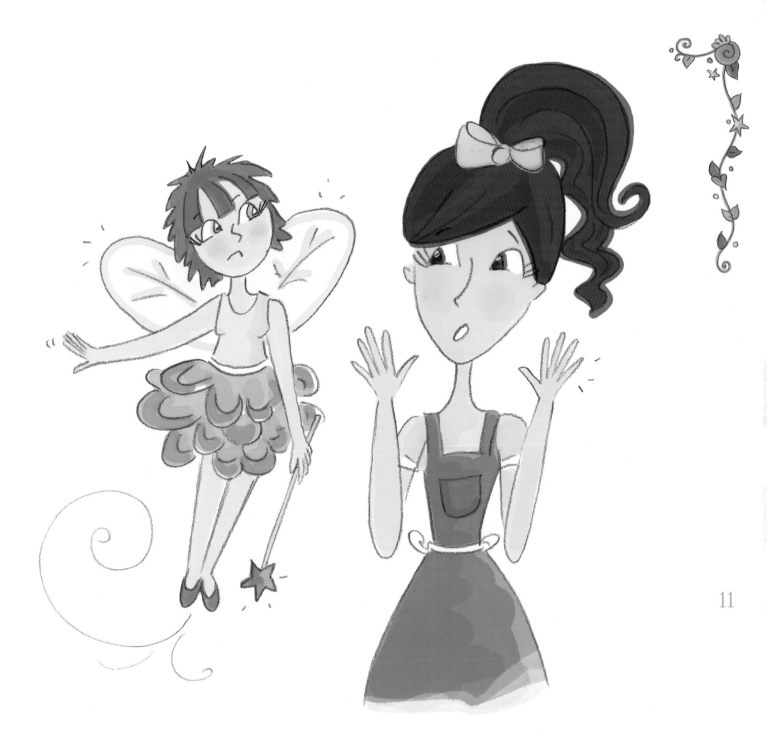

"No!" Kylie interrupted,
"Thank you, but I can't use any of those ingredients.
I'm very allergic to them.
My cookies need to be milk-,
egg-, and nut-free."

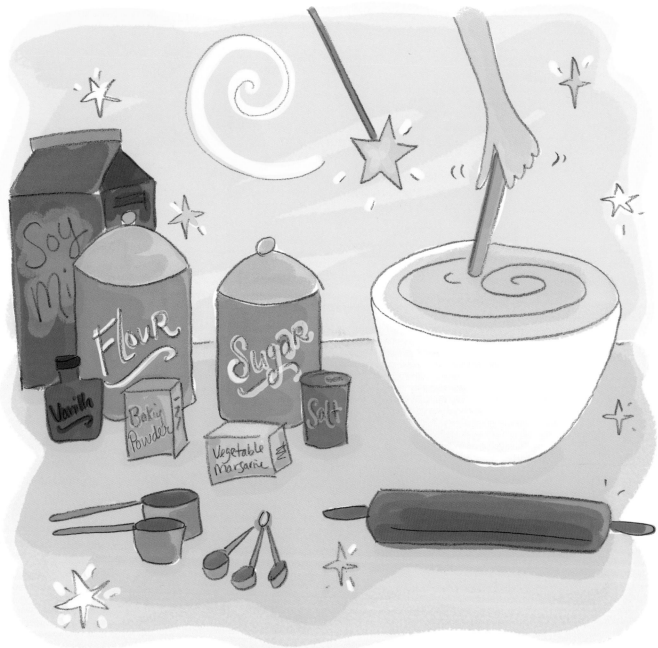

"Milk-, egg-, and nut-free sounds good to me!" said the fairy. She waved her wand, and POOF! All of Kylie's safe ingredients flew out of the cupboard and onto the table! Kylie giggled and mixed the special dough and dropped the cookies onto the baking pans.

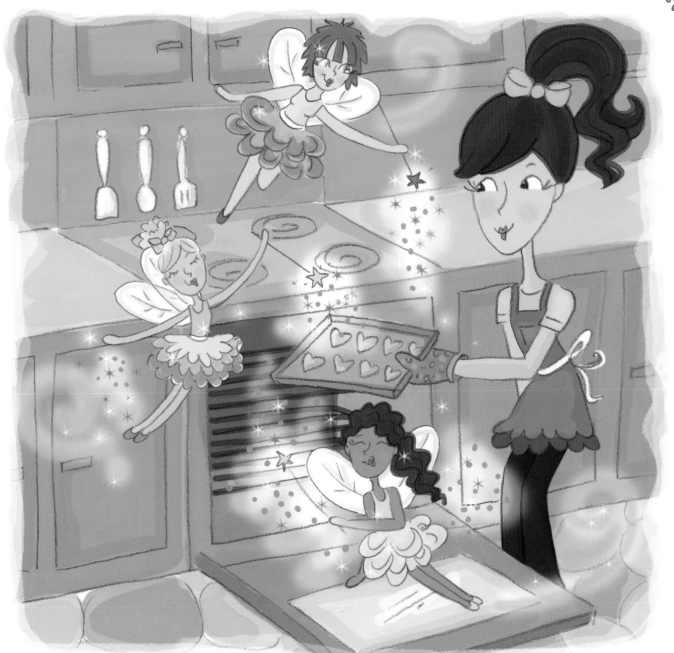

13

Just before she put the cookies in the oven,
the fairies whipped around the room and dusted
the cookies with safe and sparkling pink sprinkles.
"What a perfect finishing touch!"
Kylie said.

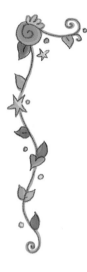

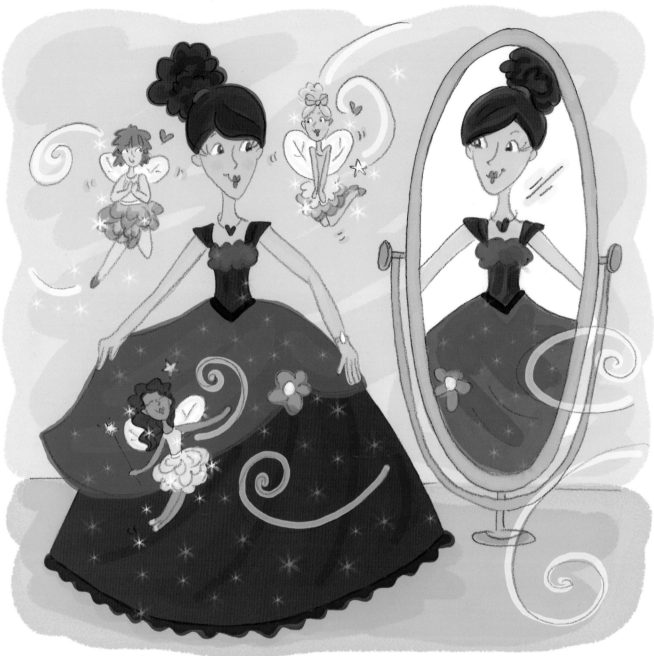

14

While Kylie got ready for the ball,
she could smell the sweet aroma of her fresh-baked goodies.
And when she looked at herself in the mirror,
she was happy to notice how her dress sparkled—
pink, like her fairy-dusted cookies.

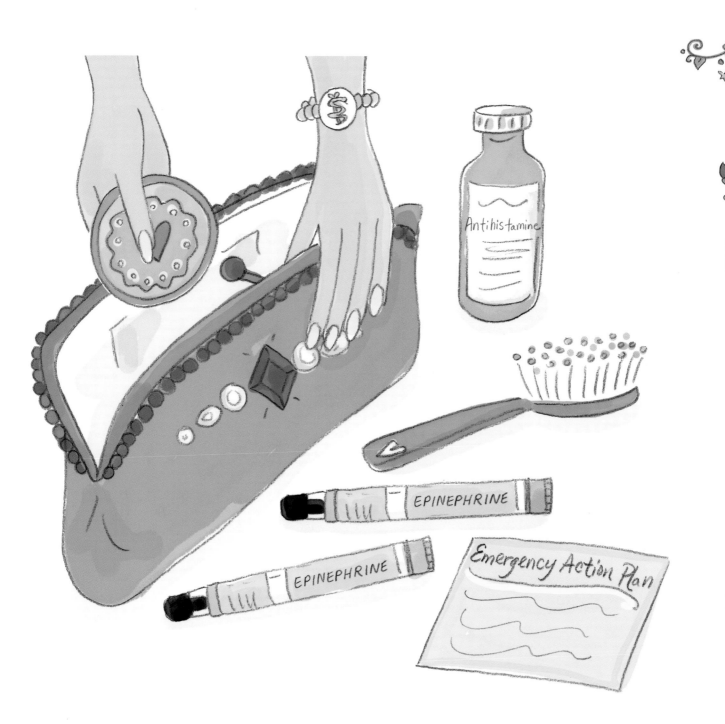

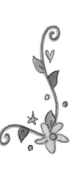

Kylie put on her medical bracelet. And, she remembered to pack her dinner. When Kylie prepares and brings her own food, she knows it is safe. In her purse she had her medicine.
If she accidentally ate or touched a food she was allergic to, she would need it! Kylie never left home without it.

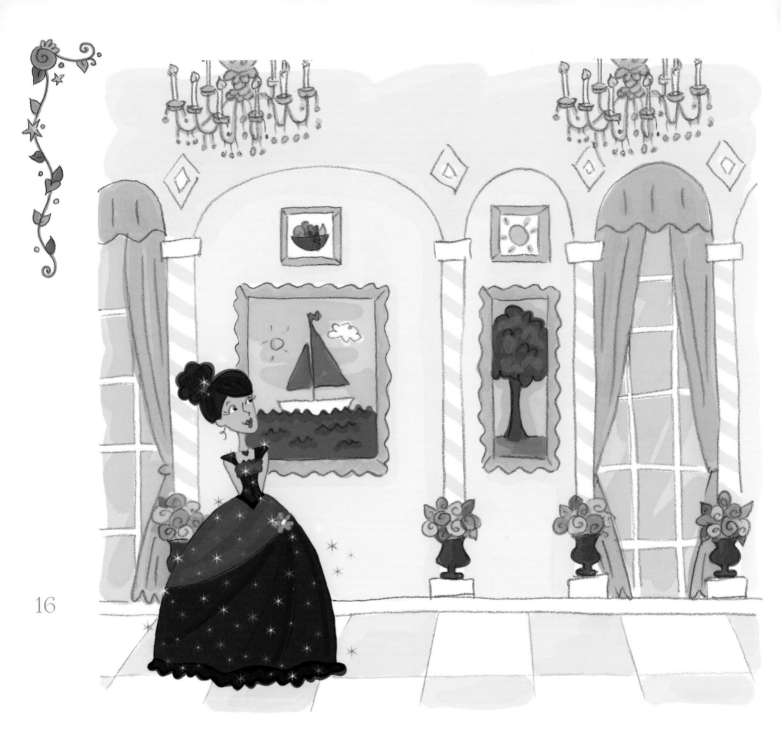

The ball was even fancier than Kylie had imagined.
The ballroom was adorned with gold chandeliers,
dangling crystals, and colorful flowers.
The walls were filled with Prince Steven's artwork.
Kylie felt so lucky to be there.

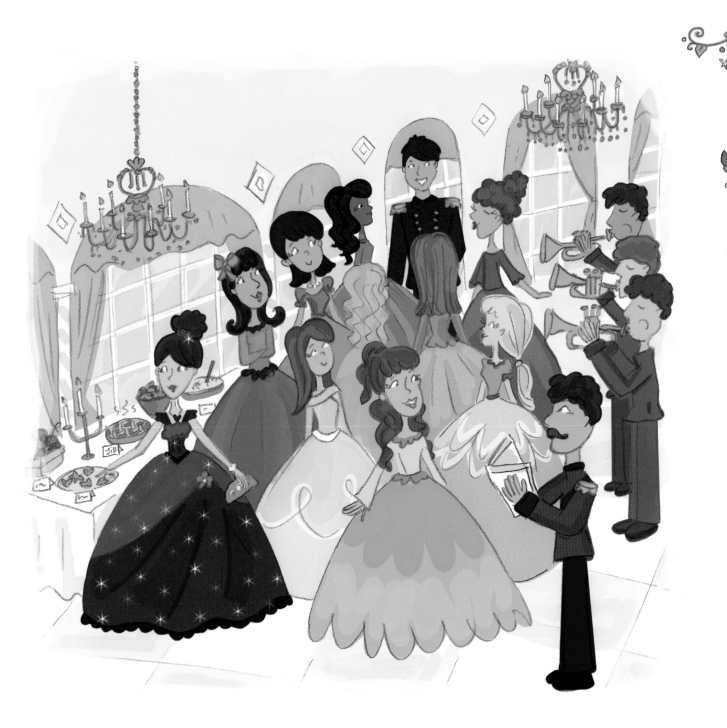

The ballroom quickly filled with many guests. The ladies carried their dishes to a long table. Each placed her dish behind a card with her name on it. Suddenly, the trumpets blared and the Grand Duke announced, "Ladies and Gentlemen of the Kingdom, Prince Steven!"

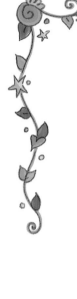

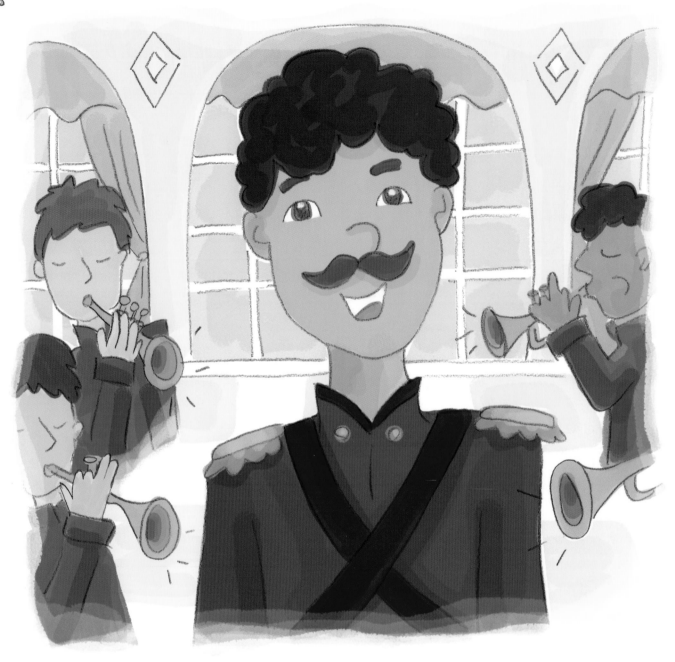

After delicious dining and dancing,
the trumpets blared again. The Grand Duke declared,
"Thank you all for coming and bringing such delectable
foods. Prince Steven has tasted each one
and will announce his favorite on Monday".

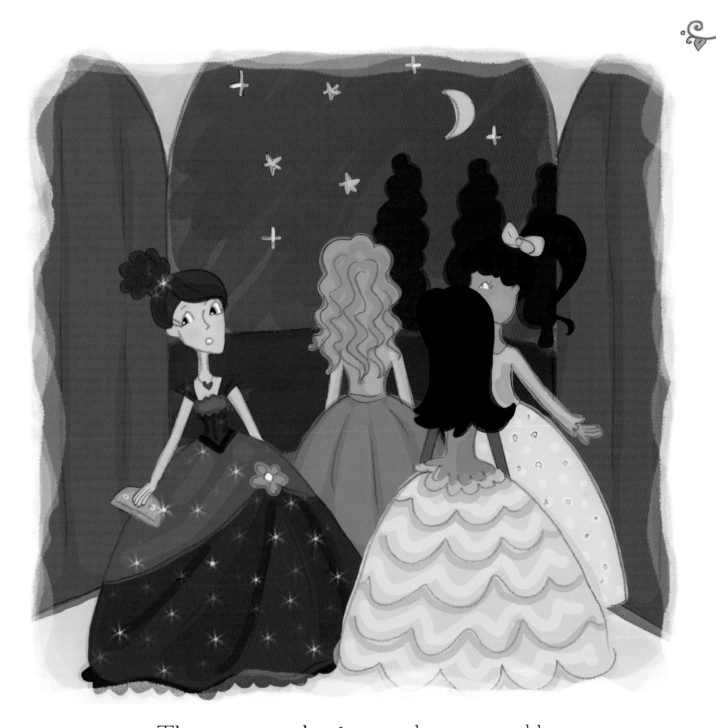

The evening had gone by so quickly.
The ball ended before Kylie had a chance
to talk to Prince Steven.
Disappointed, and without a dance,
she returned home.

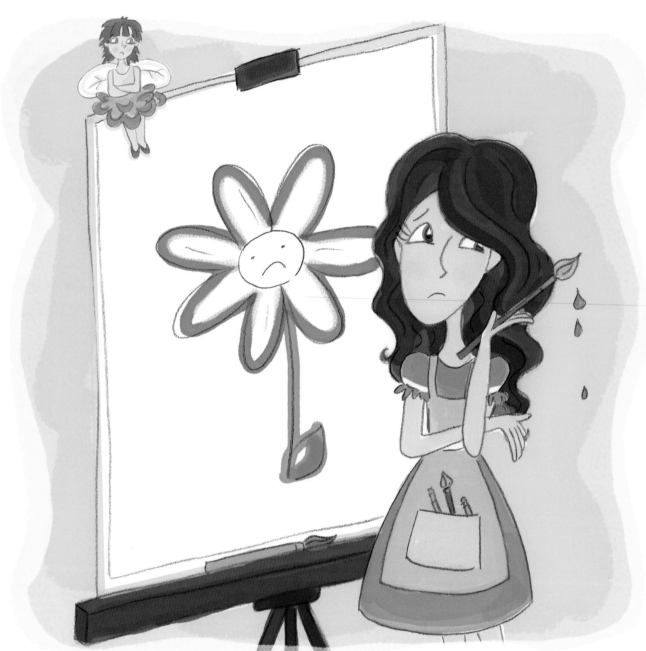

The next morning, Kylie stood at her easel,
but she did not feel like painting.
Her mind kept drifting back to the ball.
She only wished she could have spoken and danced
with Prince Steven.

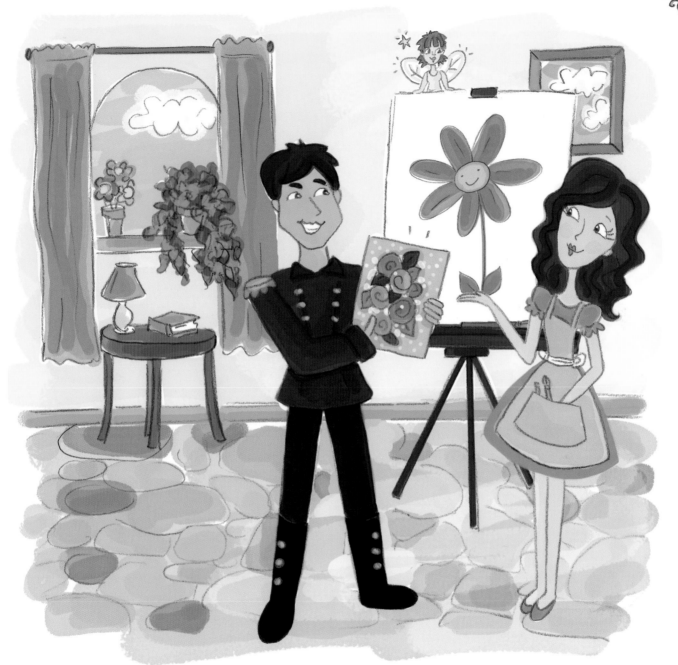

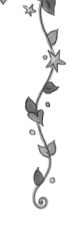

A knock at the door awoke her from her daydream.
She opened the door to Prince Steven's sparkling hazel eyes
and bright smile. "Kylie! I am so happy to see you," he said.
"I am happy to see you too!" Kylie answered.
And she saw his delight as he looked at her paintings.

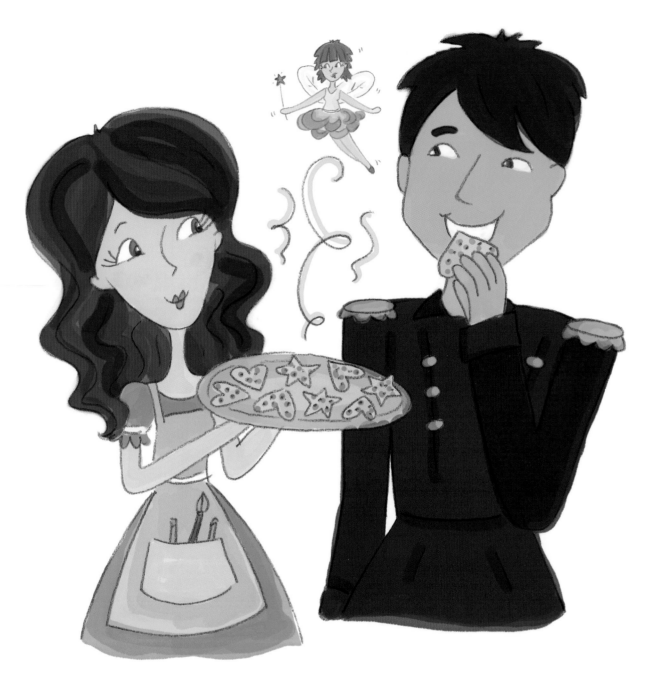

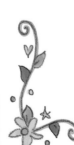

They talked about art. Kylie offered the prince a sugar cookie. "You baked these!?" he exclaimed. "The wind blew all the name cards off the table as everyone was leaving the ball. I spent the morning going house to house, searching for the person who baked these cookies!"

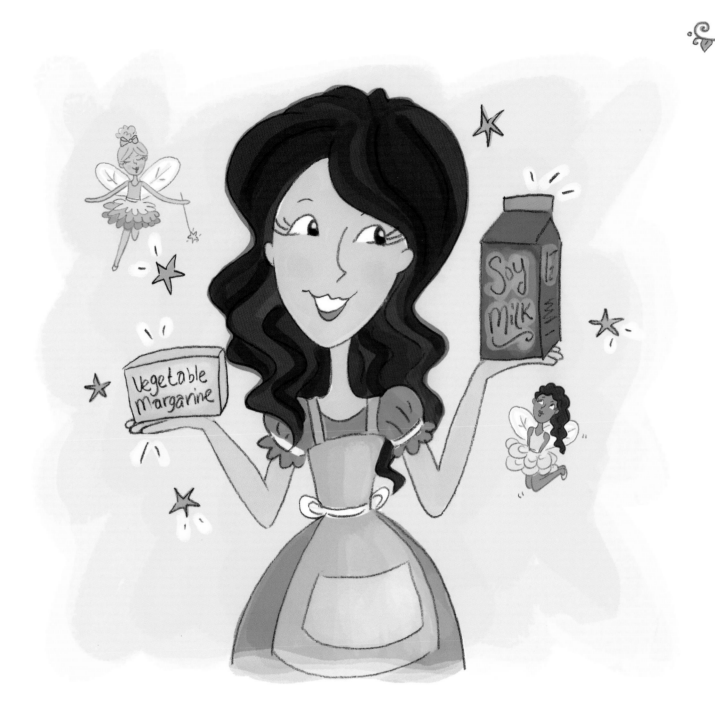

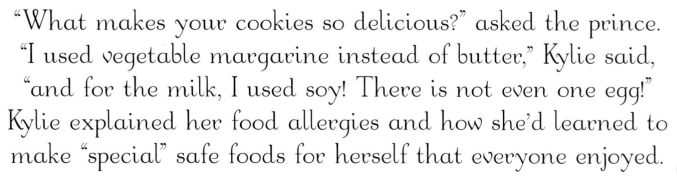

"What makes your cookies so delicious?" asked the prince.
"I used vegetable margarine instead of butter," Kylie said,
"and for the milk, I used soy! There is not even one egg!"
Kylie explained her food allergies and how she'd learned to
make "special" safe foods for herself that everyone enjoyed.

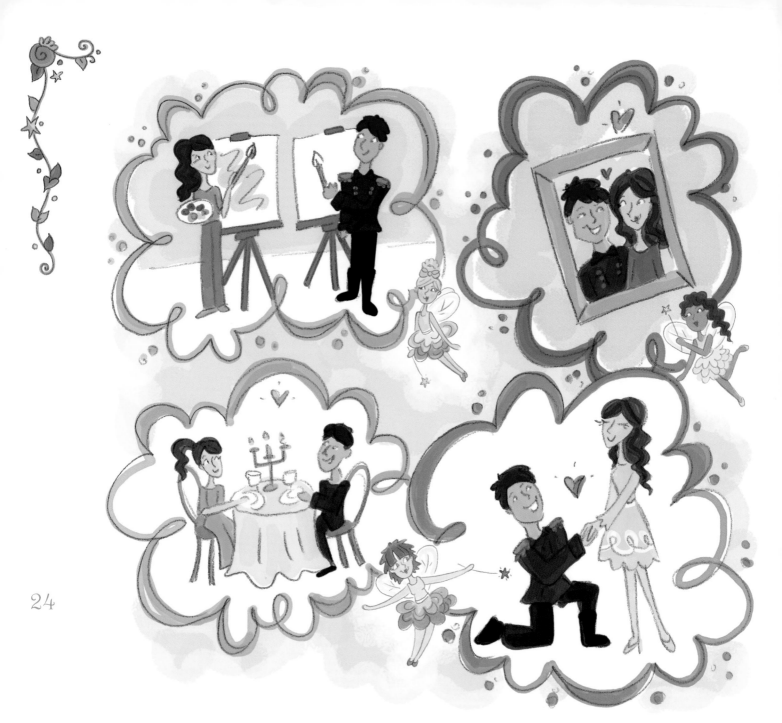

From that day forward
Kylie and Prince Steven were inseparable.
The fairies thought it was their magical pink sprinkles,
but everyone could see
that Kylie and Prince Steven were meant to be.

24

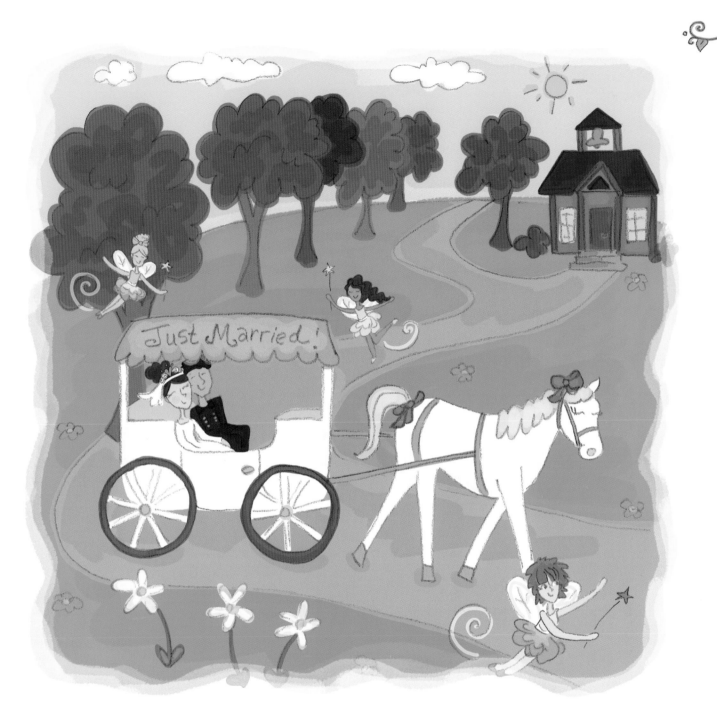

One summer afternoon, the prince asked,
"Kylie, will you marry me?"
Not only did Prince Steven and Princess Kylie
live happily ever after, but Princess Kylie and Prince Steven
opened their very own art school in the kingdom.

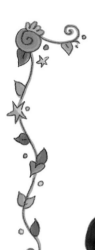

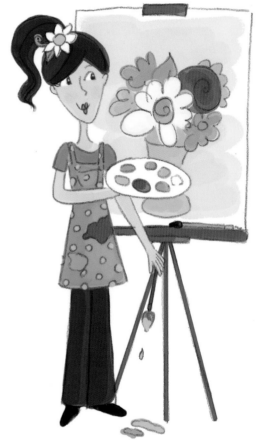

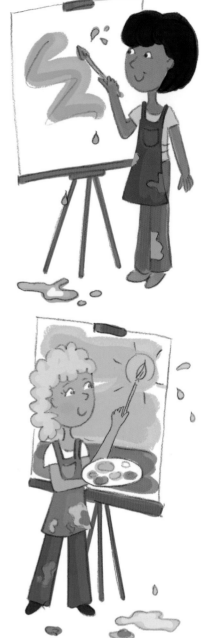

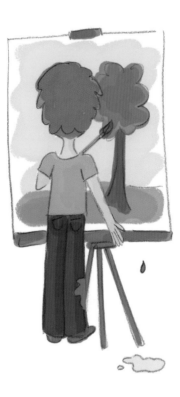

When she learned that some of her students had
food allergies too, Princess Kylie happily shared her story.
She also shared some of her special recipes
with her student's parents and, like every good teacher,
shared other tips about safety.

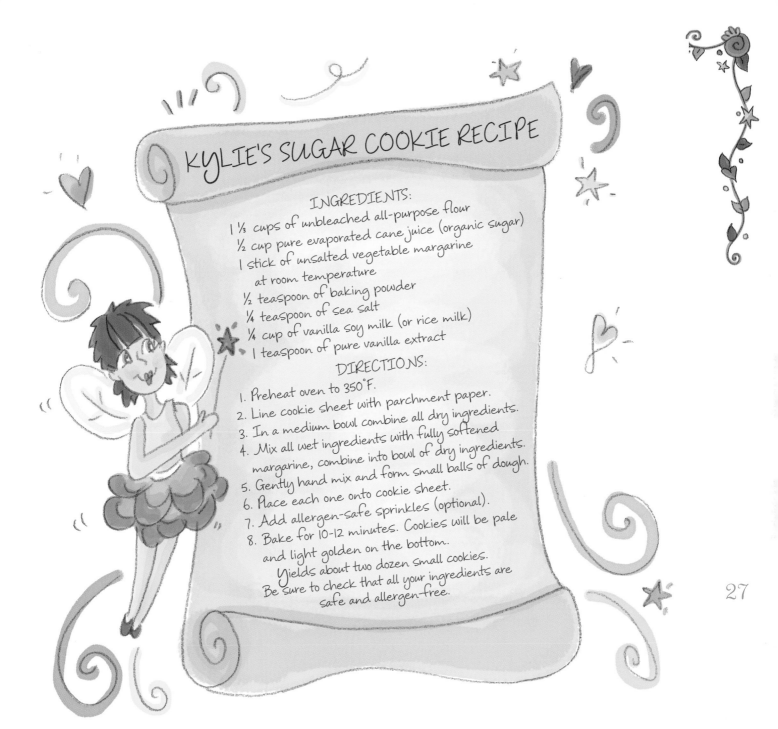

KYLIE'S SUGAR COOKIE RECIPE

INGREDIENTS:

1 ⅓ cups of unbleached all-purpose flour
½ cup pure evaporated cane juice (organic sugar)
1 stick of unsalted vegetable margarine
   at room temperature
½ teaspoon of baking powder
¼ teaspoon of sea salt
¼ cup of vanilla soy milk (or rice milk)
1 teaspoon of pure vanilla extract

DIRECTIONS:

1. Preheat oven to 350°F.
2. Line cookie sheet with parchment paper.
3. In a medium bowl combine all dry ingredients.
4. Mix all wet ingredients with fully softened
   margarine, combine into bowl of dry ingredients.
5. Gently hand mix and form small balls of dough.
6. Place each one onto cookie sheet.
7. Add allergen-safe sprinkles (optional).
8. Bake for 10-12 minutes. Cookies will be pale
   and light golden on the bottom.
      Yields about two dozen small cookies.
   Be sure to check that all your ingredients are
             safe and allergen-free.

Princess Kylie's special treat
was declared the
"Official Cookie of the Kingdom"
and everyone was given the recipe to bake
and enjoy at home with their families.

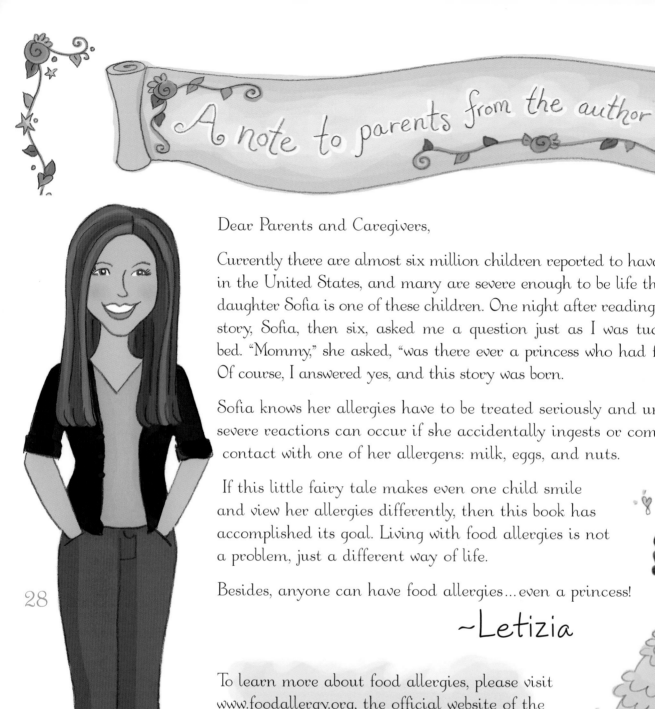

A note to parents from the author

Dear Parents and Caregivers,

Currently there are almost six million children reported to have food allergies in the United States, and many are severe enough to be life threatening. My daughter Sofia is one of these children. One night after reading her a princess story, Sofia, then six, asked me a question just as I was tucking her into bed. "Mommy," she asked, "was there ever a princess who had food allergies?" Of course, I answered yes, and this story was born.

Sofia knows her allergies have to be treated seriously and understands severe reactions can occur if she accidentally ingests or comes in contact with one of her allergens: milk, eggs, and nuts.

If this little fairy tale makes even one child smile and view her allergies differently, then this book has accomplished its goal. Living with food allergies is not a problem, just a different way of life.

Besides, anyone can have food allergies...even a princess!

~Letizia

To learn more about food allergies, please visit www.foodallergy.org, the official website of the Food Allergy and Anaphylaxis Network (FAAN). This organization's mission is to increase public awareness about food allergies and anaphylaxis, to provide education, and to advance research on behalf of all of those affected by food allergies.

A portion of the proceeds from each book sold will be donated to FAAN for food allergy research.

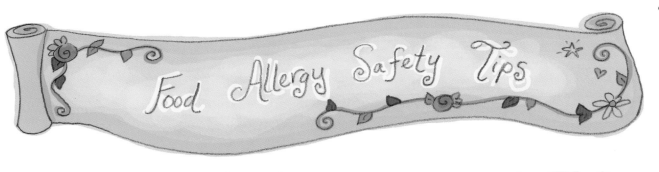

Food Allergy Safety Tips

Treat your child's medication with TLC:

"Take it... Leave it... Check it!"

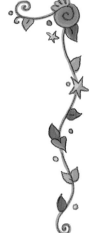

Take it: If your child has been prescribed epinephrine, be sure to take two EpiPens®, the antihistamine, and the Emergency Action Plan with you wherever you go... always!

Leave it: Leave an extra supply of your child's medicine where she spends most of her time outside of the home; for example, at school or a grandparent's house. Clearly print her name on a medicine bag (or a large ziplock bag) and include all necessary medication inside along with a copy of her Emergency Action Plan, complete with phone numbers. Teach the person in charge what symptoms to look for and the right way to treat a possible reaction, as well as how to administer the medicine.

29

Check it! Check the expiration dates of both the antihistamine medicine and the epinephrine injectors. Write the dates on your home calendar; you can even send yourself a reminder on your cell phone. If you have an EpiPen®, you can visit the manufacturer's website at www.MyEpiPen.com and register each EpiPen® so you will receive an email notification about its expiration date.

Download a full list of helpful tips at
www.PrincessWithFoodAllergies.com

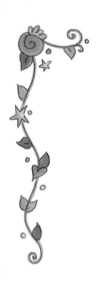

30

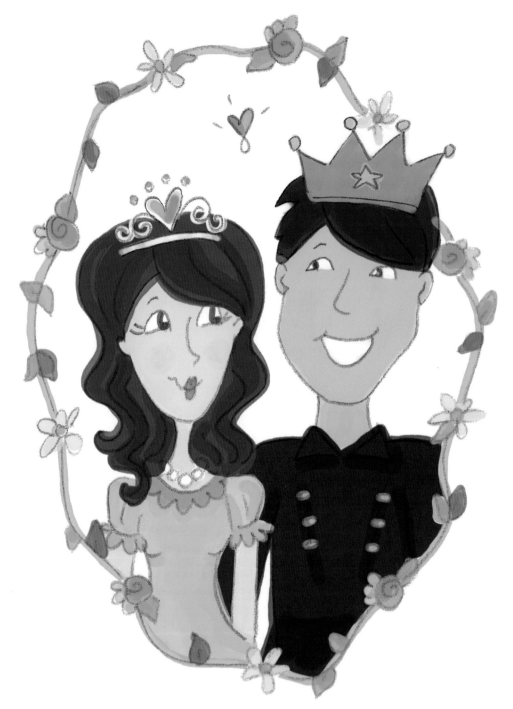

Meet Princess Kylie online! Share your own story with her, get her favorite
allergy-free recipes, download extra safety tips and fun coloring pages:
www.PrincessWithFoodAllergies.com

...and let's live happily ever after!

Food Allergy Resources

Websites

KidsWithFoodAllergies.org
AllergyReady.com
AllergyMoms.com

Books

Caring for Your Child with Severe Food Allergies
Lisa Cipriano Collins, M.A., M.F.T.

The Food Allergy Mama's Baking Book
Kelly Rudnicki

Food Allergies for Dummies®
Robert A. Wood, MD with Joe Kraynak

Magazines

Allergic Living
Living Without®
Allergy & Asthma Today

Get more resources online at:
www.PrincessWithFoodAllergies.com

www..com

$ 18.95